AF866341

Preface

I still remember what it felt like to finish my PMHNP program.

Years of hard work had finally led to this moment. I had earned the degree, passed the boards, and was ready to begin the career I had worked so hard to achieve.

Then reality set in.

Like many new Psychiatric-Mental Health Nurse Practitioners, I quickly realized that graduation was not the finish line—it was the starting line.

My education gave me a strong foundation in psychiatric assessment, psychopharmacology, psychotherapy, and evidence-based practice. It taught me how to think critically and care for patients safely. But no classroom can fully prepare you for the responsibility of sitting across from a patient who is looking to you for answers. No textbook can completely teach the clinical judgment that develops through experience. And no examination can measure the confidence that is earned one patient encounter at a time.

During my early years in practice, I discovered that becoming a competent clinician was about far more than knowing medications or diagnostic criteria. It was learning how to manage uncertainty. It was recognizing what I did not know and having the humility to seek guidance. Most importantly, it was learning that the best providers never stop learning.

One of the greatest lessons I learned is that no one succeeds alone. Throughout my journey, I was fortunate to be surrounded by people who generously shared their knowledge and encouraged my growth. Even after graduating, I continued to seek guidance from the preceptors who trained me during my PMHNP program. I stayed connected with the psychiatrists I had the privilege of working with when I was a registered nurse, whose clinical wisdom shaped the way I approach patient care today. I leaned on my fellow nurses from the psychiatric hospital where I worked, whose experience and practical insights reminded me that healthcare is always a team effort. I also remained close to many of my classmates from nurse practitioner school.

Those relationships became one of the greatest assets of my professional career. They reminded me that asking for help is not a sign of weakness—it is a hallmark of professionalism. Even today, after years in practice, teaching and precepting, doing research and participating in clinical trials, and starting a practice and expanding it to seven offices and in three states, I continue to learn from colleagues, mentors, other practice owners, students, and the patients who place their trust in me.

As an immigrant, communication was not always easy for me. English was not my first language, and there were times when expressing my thoughts felt more difficult than understanding the science itself. Over time, I learned that patients do not expect perfection. They value honesty, compassion, respect, and someone who genuinely listens. Those qualities matter just as much as clinical knowledge.

Throughout my career, I have had the privilege of serving in many roles—as a clinician, educator, researcher, speaker, and entrepreneur. Each role has reinforced the same lesson: our profession is built on lifelong learning.

As I began teaching and mentoring PMHNP and medical students, I noticed a common theme. Nearly everyone asked the same questions.
"Am I ready?"
"What if I miss something?"
"How do experienced providers make these decisions?"
"Will I ever feel confident?"

The answer is yes—but confidence does not appear overnight. It develops gradually through preparation, reflection, experience, and the willingness to keep learning.

That realization is why I wrote this book.

This is not another psychopharmacology textbook. It is not a board review manual. It is not intended to replace your clinical guidelines, experienced colleagues, or continuing education.

Instead, think of this book as a conversation with a mentor.

If we were sitting together after clinic, these are the lessons I would share with you. The practical advice I wish someone had given me. The mistakes to avoid. The habits that build confidence.

Throughout these pages, you will find clinical pearls, practical strategies, reflective questions, and real-world insights drawn from years of patient care, teaching, mentorship, and leadership. My hope is not to give you every answer—because no single book can do that. My goal is to help you develop the mindset and clinical reasoning that will guide you throughout your career.

Medicine evolves, psychiatry evolves, and we must evolve with it. Psychiatry is a remarkable specialty. We are invited into people's lives during some of their most vulnerable moments. While the responsibility can feel overwhelming at times, it is also one of the greatest privileges in healthcare.

As you begin this journey, remember that you are not expected to know everything. None of us did when we started. Build your network of mentors. Value the wisdom of experienced nurses, physicians, therapists, pharmacists, and fellow nurse practitioners. Never hesitate to ask questions, seek another perspective, or admit when you need help. The strongest clinicians are not those who know everything—they are those who are committed to learning every day.

I hope this guide becomes a trusted companion during your first months and years in practice—a reminder that every experienced PMHNP was once exactly where you are today.

Welcome to the lifelong journey of becoming an exceptional Psychiatric Mental Health Nurse Practitioner.

Liberty Olive RB Macias, DNP, APRN, PMHNP-BC

Chapter 1
Congratulations… You are a PMHNP. Now What?

"Success is not the end of your education—it is the beginning of your responsibility."

Before you update your résumé, apply for jobs, or prepare for your first day in clinic, pause and appreciate what you have accomplished.

You completed graduate school, survived clinical rotations, passed your board certification, and earned the privilege of calling yourself a Psychiatric Mental Health Nurse Practitioner. That achievement represents years of sacrifice, perseverance, and hard work.

Now begins one of the most rewarding and humbling chapters of your professional life.

From this day forward, patients, families, and colleagues will trust you to help navigate some of life's most difficult moments. That is both an incredible privilege and a tremendous responsibility.

The Feeling No One Talks About

Many new graduates expect confidence to arrive the moment they become licensed.

It usually does not.

Instead, you may find yourself wondering:

> *"Am I really ready?"*
> *"What if I miss something?"*
> *"What if I make the wrong decision?"*

If you have had these thoughts, you are not alone. Every experienced PMHNP has stood exactly where you are today.
Confidence is not something you receive with your diploma.
It is built one patient, one decision, and one lesson at a time.

School Gave You the Foundation

Your PMHNP program gave you something far more valuable than memorized facts. It taught you how to assess patients, think critically, develop differential diagnoses, evaluate evidence, and practice safely.

Those skills are your foundation.

Your first year of practice is where that foundation begins to transform into clinical judgment. You will recognize patterns, become more efficient, and gain confidence through experience. Every patient will teach you something new.

Remember, no educational program can prepare you for every clinical situation. Psychiatry is complex because every patient is unique.

Your First Year Matters

Your first year is not about becoming the perfect clinician.

It is about becoming a better clinician every day.

You will spend extra time reviewing medications, reading practice guidelines, and double-checking treatment plans. You will probably think of the perfect follow-up question after your patient has already left the office. You may rewrite your documentation more than once before signing it.

That is normal.

Growth in psychiatry does not happen overnight. It develops through experience, reflection, and the humility to continue asking questions.

You Don't Have to Know Everything

One of the greatest lessons you will learn is that good clinicians do not have every answer.

They know how to ask the right questions.

They know where to find reliable information.
And they know when to seek another opinion.

Psychiatry continues to evolve. New research, medications, and treatment guidelines emerge every year. Your greatest strength will never be knowing everything—it will be your commitment to lifelong learning and providing thoughtful, evidence-based care.

Patients do not expect perfection.

They expect honesty, compassion, and someone who genuinely cares about helping them.

Never underestimate the power of simply listening.

Looking Ahead
The chapters that follow are designed to help you navigate the transition from graduate to practicing clinician. We will discuss preparing for your first job, conducting psychiatric evaluations, prescribing with confidence, documenting effectively, protecting your license, and building a meaningful career.

My goal is not to teach you everything about psychiatry.

My goal is to help you think like a psychiatric clinician.

Mentor's Corner
You earned your place here.

Be curious.

Stay humble.

Ask questions.

Continue learning.

Those qualities will take you much farther than trying to appear as though you have all the answers.

Quick Checklist
Before you see your first patient, ask yourself:
- ✓ *Have I identified mentors I can reach out to when I have questions?*
- ✓ *Do I know where to find current clinical guidelines, prescribing resources, and trusted references?*
- ✓ *Have I committed to lifelong learning rather than expecting immediate mastery?*
- ✓ *Am I willing to ask for help when I need it?*
- ✓ *Am I prepared to treat every patient with curiosity, humility, and compassion?*

If you answered "yes" to these questions, you are already thinking like a PMHNP.

Liberty's Lesson #1
The day you think you no longer need mentors is the day your professional growth begins to slow.

Stay connected with the people who helped shape your journey. Keep in touch with your preceptors. Reach out to former colleagues. Build relationships with psychiatrists, therapists, psychologists, pharmacists, nurses, and fellow nurse practitioners. Discuss difficult cases. Celebrate successes. Learn from one another.

Psychiatry is too complex to practice in isolation, and the best clinicians never stop seeking wisdom from others.

Your degree made you a PMHNP. Your willingness to keep learning will make you an exceptional one.

Chapter 2
Preparing For Practice

"Preparation builds confidence long before your first patient walks through the door."

Whether you are joining a private practice, community mental health clinic, hospital, telepsychiatry group, or opening your own practice, taking time to prepare will make your transition smoother and less stressful.

You do not need to have every answer before you start—but you should have the right tools, resources, and habits in place.

Get Your Professional House in Order

Before seeing patients, make sure you have completed the essentials:

- Active APRN and RN licenses
- Board certification
- DEA registration (if applicable)
- National Provider Identifier (NPI)
- State controlled substance registration (if required)
- Malpractice insurance
- Credentialing and payer enrollment
- Employment paperwork and compliance training

These tasks may not be exciting, but they are the foundation of safe and legal practice.

Know Your Resources

No clinician practices from memory alone.

Experienced providers regularly consult trusted references, clinical guidelines, and prescribing resources.

Before your first day, identify the resources you will rely on, such as:

- Current psychiatric treatment guidelines
- A reliable drug reference
- Drug interaction checker
- Laboratory interpretation resources
- Prescription monitoring program (PDMP)
- Your organization's policies and protocols

Know your resources before you need them.

Learn Your Workplace

Every practice has its own workflow.

Take time to understand:

- The electronic health record (EHR)
- Documentation expectations
- Prescription processes
- Prior authorization procedures
- Referral pathways
- Crisis protocols
- Emergency contacts
- After-hours responsibilities

Knowing how your clinic functions allows you to focus on your patients instead of scrambling to find answers.

Find Your People

One of the smartest things you can do is identify experienced colleagues you can learn from.

Ask questions.

Observe how they approach difficult cases.

Discuss treatment decisions.

Request feedback.

Remember, mentorship does not end with graduation. It evolves throughout your career.

Create a Learning Routine

The most successful PMHNPs do not try to learn everything in one weekend. Instead, they build consistent habits.

Consider setting aside time each week to:

- Read one journal article.
- Review one treatment guideline.
- Learn about one medication.
- Reflect on one challenging patient.
- Discuss one case with a colleague or mentor.

Small, consistent efforts lead to lasting growth.

Prepare Yourself, Not Just Your Office
Clinical knowledge is important, but so is your mindset.

Your patients do not need you to be perfect.
They need you to be present.
Listen carefully.

Treat every patient with dignity.

Never be afraid to say, "Let me review that and get back to you."
Patients appreciate honesty far more than false confidence.

Looking Ahead
You have prepared your workspace.
You have organized your resources.

Now it is time to focus on the most important part of psychiatric practice:
The patient interview.

In the next chapter, we will discuss how to approach your first psychiatric evaluation with confidence, curiosity, and clinical reasoning.

Mentor's Corner
Preparation reduces anxiety.
The better prepared you are before clinic begins, the more mental energy you will have to focus on what truly matters—your patients.

Quick Checklist
Before your first day, make sure you can answer "yes" to these questions:

- ✓ *Are my licenses, certifications, and registrations complete?*
- ✓ *Do I know how to use my organization's* EHR*?*
- ✓ *Do I know where to find treatment guidelines and drug references?*
- ✓ *Do I understand the clinic's workflow and emergency procedures?*
- ✓ *Have I identified at least one experienced clinician I can turn to with questions?*
- ✓ *Do I have a plan for continuing my learning every week?*

Liberty's Lesson #2
Never confuse preparation with weakness.

Early in my career, I spent extra time reviewing charts, reading treatment guidelines, and double-checking medication decisions before seeing patients.
At times, I wondered if that meant I was not ready.

Preparation is not a sign that you lack confidence—it is a sign that you take your responsibility seriously.

The clinicians I respect most still prepare before clinic. They review difficult cases, stay current with the literature, and continue learning long after training has ended.

The goal is not to become the fastest provider in the room.
The goal is to become a thoughtful, safe, and trusted one.

Chapter 3
Thinking Like a Psychiatric Provider

"Knowledge tells you what could be happening. Clinical reasoning helps you determine what is happening."

One of the biggest transitions you will make as a new PMHNP is not learning more psychiatry—it is learning to think differently.

As a student, much of your focus was on finding the correct answer. Exams often had one best choice, and textbooks presented disorders in neat categories.

Real patients rarely do.
They do not walk into your office saying, "I have major depressive disorder."
Instead, they may say:
"I'm exhausted."
"I can't sleep."
"My family says I'm different."
"I'm having panic attacks."

Your job is to uncover the story behind those symptoms.

Slow Down Before You Diagnose

One of the most common mistakes new clinicians make is deciding on a diagnosis too early.

Perhaps the patient says they are depressed, and you immediately think, "Major depressive disorder."

But experienced clinicians pause.
They ask:
Could this be bipolar disorder?
Is substance use contributing?
Could there be a medical condition?
Is this grief, trauma, or an adjustment disorder?
What information am I still missing?

The best diagnosis is rarely the fastest one.

Think in Differentials

Every patient deserves a thoughtful differential diagnosis.

Rather than asking, *"What's the diagnosis?"* ask yourself:
"What are the most likely possibilities, and what evidence supports or argues against each one?"

Keeping an open mind reduces the risk of premature conclusions and helps ensure your treatment plan is based on careful clinical reasoning.

Treat the Patient, Not the Label

Psychiatric diagnoses are important, but patients are more than diagnostic criteria.

Two people with the same diagnosis may have very different experiences, goals, medical histories, and treatment preferences.

Listen carefully.
Understand what matters most to your patient.

A diagnosis guides treatment, but the person in front of you should always guide your care.

Learn to Be Comfortable With Uncertainty

Not every patient will fit neatly into a diagnostic category during the first visit.
Sometimes the most appropriate plan is to gather more information, obtain collateral history, review previous records, or schedule close follow-up.
Remember, psychiatry often unfolds over time.

Every Encounter Is an Opportunity to Learn

No matter how experienced you become, every patient will teach you something.

Some will reinforce what you already know.
Others will challenge your assumptions.

Read after clinic.
Review the evidence.
Discuss difficult cases with trusted colleagues.
The clinicians who continue growing are the ones who never stop asking questions.

Looking Ahead

Now that we have discussed how psychiatric clinicians think, it is time to apply that mindset.
In the next chapter, we will walk through the psychiatric evaluation—from building rapport and gathering information to developing a thoughtful assessment and treatment plan.

Mentor's Corner

Do not rush to prove that you are knowledgeable.
Instead, demonstrate that you are thoughtful.

Patients benefit far more from a clinician who listens carefully than one who reaches conclusions too quickly.

Quick Checklist
Before finalizing your assessment, ask yourself:

- ✓ *Have I considered more than one possible diagnosis?*
- ✓ *Is there a medical, neurological, or substance-related explanation?*
- ✓ *Do I have enough information to support my diagnosis?*
- ✓ *Am I treating the patient as a whole person, not just a diagnosis?*
- ✓ *What information do I still need?*

Liberty's Lesson #3
Your first diagnosis does not have to be your final diagnosis.

Early in practice, I learned that psychiatry rewards curiosity more than certainty. Some diagnoses become clearer only after trust has been established, additional history is obtained, or symptoms evolve over time.

Never feel pressured to force a diagnosis simply because you think you need an answer today.

Patients are best served when we remain open-minded, continue gathering information, and allow the clinical picture to unfold.

Sometimes the most thoughtful decision you can make is to say, **"I need to learn a little more before I label this."**

Clinical Reasoning in Action
The Patient Who "Just Needed an Antidepressant"

Maria, a 34-year-old elementary school teacher, was referred by her primary care provider for depression. She described feeling exhausted, unmotivated, and unable to enjoy activities she once loved. Her PHQ-9 score was 18, and she asked if she could "just start an antidepressant."

At first glance, Major Depressive Disorder seemed like the obvious diagnosis. Instead of immediately discussing medication, you continued the interview.

You asked about previous mood episodes, sleep patterns, family psychiatric history, substance use, medical conditions, and recent stressors.

Maria then shared that every few months she experienced periods lasting three to four days when she slept only a few hours each night, felt unusually productive, became more talkative than usual, and started ambitious projects she rarely finished. She laughed and said, "I always thought those were my good days."

She also mentioned that an aunt had been diagnosed with bipolar disorder. The interview suddenly took a different direction.

Reflection Questions

Before reading further, consider the following:

What additional questions would you ask?
What diagnoses should remain on your differential?
Would you start an antidepressant today? Why or why not?
What additional information would help you make a safe treatment decision?

How I Would Think Through This Case

The patient's current symptoms are certainly consistent with a depressive episode, but experienced clinicians resist the urge to stop there.

Her history raises several important considerations: episodes of decreased need for sleep, increased energy, impulsive behavior, and a family history of bipolar disorder. These findings warrant a more thorough assessment for Bipolar II Disorder before initiating treatment.

Rather than rushing to prescribe an antidepressant, I would continue gathering history, review previous records if available, assess current safety, and discuss the importance of making an accurate diagnosis before selecting medication.

A few extra minutes of thoughtful questioning may prevent years of inappropriate treatment.

Clinical Pearl: The most important prescription you write is the correct diagnosis

Chapter 4
Meeting Your First Patient

"Patients may not remember every medication you prescribed, but they will remember how you made them feel."

Walking into your first appointment as a PMHNP can be intimidating.
You have reviewed the chart. You have rehearsed the questions in your mind. You remind yourself of the DSM-5-TR criteria and treatment guidelines.

Then your patient walks in.
At that moment, your greatest asset is not your memory or your knowledge of psychopharmacology.
It is your ability to connect with another human being.

Start with the Person, Not the Chart
Charts tell you what has been documented.
Patients tell you what has been lived.

Although reviewing the medical record before entering the room is important, do not let it create tunnel vision. Previous diagnoses may be incomplete, outdated, or even incorrect.

Approach every evaluation with curiosity.

One of my favorite questions to begin an interview is:
"Tell me what brought you in today."

Then listen.
Allow the patient to tell their story before directing the interview. Often, the first few uninterrupted minutes provide valuable information about their concerns, priorities, and communication style.

Build Rapport Before Gathering Information
A successful psychiatric interview is more than a checklist of symptoms.
Patients are often sharing deeply personal experiences—sometimes for the very first time.

Simple actions can make a meaningful difference:

- Introduce yourself clearly.
- Explain your role.
- Maintain eye contact.
- Avoid interrupting unnecessarily.
- Use language your patient understands.
- Normalize difficult conversations when appropriate.

Patients are more likely to share sensitive information when they feel respected and heard.

Be Curious, Not Curious to Confirm

One of the easiest traps for new clinicians is confirmation bias—the tendency to look only for information that supports your first impression.

Instead, challenge yourself to ask:
"What else could explain these symptoms?"

Remain open to alternative diagnoses throughout the interview.
Sometimes the most important information is revealed during the last few minutes of the visit.

Listen for the Story Behind the Symptoms

Symptoms rarely exist in isolation.

As you listen, think beyond the diagnosis.
Ask yourself:

- When did this begin?
- Why now?
- What changed?
- How is this affecting daily life?
- What strengths has this patient already demonstrated?

Understanding the patient's story often explains why symptoms developed and helps guide treatment.

Do Not Forget Safety

Every psychiatric evaluation should include an assessment of safety.

Depending on the clinical situation, this may include:

- Suicidal thoughts
- Self-harm behaviors
- Homicidal thoughts
- Psychosis
- Substance use
- Access to lethal means
- Ability to care for basic needs

Risk assessment should be thoughtful and individualized—not simply a series of required questions.

End with a Shared Plan
Before concluding the visit, summarize what you have heard.
Confirm that you have understood the patient's concerns.

Discuss your assessment and recommendations in language the patient can understand.
Invite questions.

Patients are more likely to follow a treatment plan they helped create.

Looking Ahead
Now that you have completed the evaluation, it is time to answer the question every new PMHNP eventually faces:
"Which treatment should I choose?"

In the next chapter, we will discuss how to approach medication decisions thoughtfully and safely.

Mentor's Corner
The interview is not about proving how much you know.
It is about understanding the person sitting in front of you.
Patients do not care how many diagnostic criteria you can recite.
They care whether you listened.

Quick Checklist
Before ending every initial evaluation, ask yourself:

- ✓ *Did I allow the patient to tell their story?*
- ✓ *Did I consider more than one diagnosis?*
- ✓ *Did I complete an appropriate safety assessment?*
- ✓ *Did I explain my assessment in understandable language?*
- ✓ *Did the patient leave knowing the next step?*

Liberty's Lesson #4
The patient is always more important than the diagnosis.

Early in my career, I realized that two patients with the same diagnosis could require completely different approaches. One might need medication. Another might first need sleep, safety, housing, or simply someone willing to listen without judgment.

Never become so focused on finding the diagnosis that you stop seeing the person.

When patients feel respected, heard, and understood, you have already begun treatment—even before writing the first prescription.

Clinical Reasoning in Action
"I Don't Think I Need to Be Here."

A 19-year-old college student arrives for an evaluation after being encouraged by his parents to seek treatment. He sits with his arms crossed and says, "I'm only here because they made me come."

His chart lists anxiety and depression. His PHQ-9 score is elevated, but he answers most of your questions with one or two words.

You could move quickly through your checklist.
Instead, you pause.

You acknowledge that coming to a psychiatric appointment was not his idea and thank him for showing up. You ask, "If there was one thing you wish people understood about what you have been going through, what would it be?"

For the first time, he looks up.
The conversation changes.

Reflection Questions
How would you establish rapport with this patient?
What assumptions might you be making based on the referral?
How might the interview differ if you focused first on the patient's goals instead of the referral diagnosis?
What would help this patient feel heard?

How I Would Think Through This Case
Before gathering diagnostic information, I would focus on engagement.

This patient has not yet agreed that he needs treatment. Building trust is more important than completing every screening question in the first few minutes.

By acknowledging his perspective and inviting him to share his own story, I increase the likelihood of obtaining meaningful information and developing a collaborative treatment plan.

Clinical Pearl: Rapport is not separate from the psychiatric evaluation—it is one of your most important diagnostic tools.

Chapter 5
Choosing the Right Treatment

"The best treatment plan is not always the one with the most prescriptions—it is the one that best fits the patient."

After completing your psychiatric evaluation, one question naturally follows:
"What's the best treatment for this patient?"

For many new PMHNPs, this is where uncertainty begins.
Should you prescribe medication today?
Should you recommend psychotherapy first?
Do you need additional information before making a decision?
Should you refer the patient to another specialist?

These questions are part of good clinical practice.
Thoughtful clinicians pause before acting.

Start with the Diagnosis

Every treatment plan begins with the best diagnosis you can make based on the available information.

If you are uncertain about the diagnosis, it may be appropriate to gather additional history, obtain collateral information, review previous records, or schedule close follow-up before initiating treatment.

A careful diagnosis remains the foundation of effective treatment.

Many new PMHNPs feel pressured to prescribe quickly—sometimes by patients, sometimes by employers, and often by themselves.

You may feel that every appointment should end with a prescription because that is what patients expect or because you do not want them to leave disappointed.

Resist that pressure.

Thoughtful psychiatric care is not measured by how quickly you prescribe. It is measured by how carefully you evaluate, how thoughtfully you develop a treatment plan, and how safely you care for your patients.

Sometimes the best decision is to prescribe medication. Sometimes the best decision is to gather more information, obtain collateral history, review previous records, recommend psychotherapy, address substance use, or schedule close follow-up before initiating treatment.

Never confuse speed with competence.

The most respected clinicians are rarely the fastest—they are the ones whose patients know that every decision is made with careful thought and genuine concern for their well-being.

Treat the Whole Person

Two patients with the same diagnosis may require very different treatment plans.

Before deciding on medication, consider:

- *The patient's goals and preferences*
- *Symptom severity*
- *Safety concerns*
- *Medical conditions*
- *Current medications*
- *Pregnancy or reproductive considerations*
- *Substance use*
- *Previous treatment response*
- *Family history of medication response*
- *Access to psychotherapy and community resources*

Psychiatric care is never one-size-fits-all.

Medication Is Only One Tool

As PMHNPs, we prescribe medications—but medications are only one part of comprehensive psychiatric care.

Depending on the patient, your treatment plan may also include:

- Psychotherapy
- Sleep hygiene
- Exercise and nutrition
- Substance use treatment
- Stress management
- Family involvement
- Community resources
- Collaboration with primary care or other specialists

The best treatment plan often combines several approaches.

Start Low, Go Slow—But Know When Not To

You will hear this phrase throughout your career, especially when treating older adults and medically complex patients.

It is excellent advice—but it is not a universal rule.

Some patients require more rapid titration because of symptom severity, while others benefit from a slower approach to minimize adverse effects.

Rather than memorizing slogans, learn the rationale behind your decisions. Your prescribing should always balance effectiveness with safety.

Discuss Risks and Benefits

Every medication conversation should include more than dosing instructions.

Patients deserve to understand:

- Why you are recommending the medication
- Expected benefits
- Common side effects
- Serious adverse effects
- Monitoring requirements
- Alternative treatment options
- When to call the clinic
- When to seek emergency care

Shared decision-making builds trust and improves adherence.

Plan the Follow-Up

Your responsibility does not end when the prescription is sent to the pharmacy. Every treatment plan should include a clear follow-up strategy.

Ask yourself:

- When should I reassess this patient?
- What symptoms will I monitor?
- What side effects should I watch for?
- Are laboratory tests needed?
- Does the patient understand when to contact me sooner?

Good follow-up is just as important as choosing the initial treatment.

Looking Ahead

Prescribing medication is only one part of safe psychiatric practice.

Just as important is documenting your clinical reasoning.

In the next chapter, we will discuss how documentation protects your patients, supports continuity of care, and safeguards your professional practice.

Mentor's Corner
Never prescribe simply because you feel pressured to "do something."
Sometimes the most thoughtful decision is to gather more information, educate the patient, or arrange close follow-up before starting medication.

Quick Checklist
Before finalizing your treatment plan, ask yourself:

- ✓ *Am I confident in my working diagnosis?*
- ✓ *Have I considered both medication and non-medication interventions?*
- ✓ *Does this plan reflect the patient's goals and preferences?*
- ✓ *Have I discussed risks, benefits, and alternatives?*
- ✓ *Is there a clear follow-up and monitoring plan?*

Liberty's Lesson #5
Every prescription is a conversation—not just a medication order.
Patients are placing their trust in you every time they agree to start treatment.

They deserve to understand why you are making your recommendation, what to expect, and how you will support them along the way.
Never underestimate the value of taking a few extra minutes to educate, answer questions, and invite patients into the decision-making process.

When patients understand the plan, they are more likely to follow it—and more likely to trust you when challenges arise.

Clinical Reasoning in Action
"Can You Just Refill My Medication?"

A 42-year-old man schedules an appointment requesting a refill of his antidepressant. He explains that he has been taking the medication for several years and simply needs a new prescription because he changed insurance.

His previous records are unavailable.

Rather than automatically renewing the medication, you review his psychiatric history, current symptoms, previous diagnoses, medical conditions, substance use, and current medications. During the interview, he mentions periods of decreased need for sleep, impulsive spending, and increased energy that had never been evaluated.

What initially appeared to be a routine refill becomes a more comprehensive diagnostic assessment.

Reflection Questions

What additional history would you obtain before prescribing?
Would you refill the medication today? Why or why not?
How would you explain your decision to the patient?
What are the risks of assuming that a previous diagnosis is correct?

How I Would Think Through This Case

A medication refill is not simply an administrative task—it is a clinical decision.

Although continuity of care is important, every prescription represents an opportunity to confirm the diagnosis, reassess safety, review treatment response, and identify changes that may affect management.

In this case, the history raises concerns for an underlying bipolar spectrum disorder. Before continuing treatment, I would gather additional information, assess current risks, discuss my concerns with the patient, and determine whether the existing treatment remains appropriate.

Clinical Pearl: Never let the words "refill visit" prevent you from thinking like a clinician.

Chapter 6
Documentation That Protects You

"If it wasn't documented, it didn't happen."

Documentation is one of the least exciting parts of psychiatric practice—and one of the most important.

Many new PMHNPs spend hours worrying about choosing the right medication but only minutes thinking about how to document the visit. In reality, your note tells the story of your clinical reasoning. It explains what you observed, how you reached your conclusions, and why you made the decisions you did.

Good documentation benefits everyone. It helps other healthcare professionals understand your thought process, supports continuity of care, demonstrates medical necessity, and protects both your patient and your professional license.

Document Your Thinking

A common mistake among new clinicians is documenting **what** they did without explaining **why** they did it.

For example, writing:
"Continue sertraline 50 mg daily." is incomplete.

A stronger note explains the clinical reasoning:
"Patient reports significant improvement in depressive symptoms with sertraline 50 mg daily without adverse effects. PHQ-9 decreased from 18 to 8. Will continue current dose and reassess in four weeks."

Your documentation should tell the next provider exactly how you arrived at your decision.

Be Objective

Document observations—not assumptions.

Instead of writing: *"Patient was manipulative."*

Describe what you observed:

"Patient repeatedly requested early refills despite reviewing the clinic's controlled substance policy and became frustrated when informed that an early refill could not be provided."

Objective language is more accurate, more professional, and more defensible.

Every Psychiatric Note Should Answer Four Questions

By the end of your documentation, another clinician should understand:

- Why did the patient come in today?
- What did you find?
- What clinical decisions did you make?
- What is the plan moving forward?

If those questions are answered clearly, you have likely written a useful note.

Do not Forget Risk Assessment

Risk assessment is one of the most important parts of psychiatric documentation.

When appropriate, document:

- Suicidal or homicidal ideation
- Self-harm behaviors
- Protective factors
- Risk factors
- Access to lethal means
- Safety planning
- Emergency instructions

Remember, documenting that you assessed risk is just as important as documenting the outcome of that assessment.

Quality Over Quantity

Long notes are not necessarily good notes.

Avoid copying and pasting outdated information or filling your documentation with unnecessary details that do not influence today's clinical decision.

Instead, write notes that are clear, concise, accurate, and clinically meaningful. Your goal is communication—not word count.

Review Before You Sign

Before completing your note, take a moment to review it.

Ask yourself:

Does this accurately reflect today's visit?
Would another clinician understand my reasoning?
Have I documented why I made today's treatment decisions?
Is there anything missing that I would want to know if I were seeing this patient tomorrow?

Those extra few minutes can prevent misunderstandings and improve patient care.

Looking Ahead
Documentation records what happened. Communication helps patients understand what happens next.

In the next chapter, we will discuss one of the most valuable skills in psychiatry: communicating effectively with patients and families.

Mentor's Corner
Do not write your note simply to finish your documentation.

Write it as though another clinician will read it tomorrow and continue caring for your patient.

Because one day, they probably will.

Quick Checklist
Before signing your note, ask yourself:

- ✓ Did I clearly document the patient's concerns?
- ✓ Did I explain my assessment and clinical reasoning?
- ✓ Did I document risk assessment when appropriate?
- ✓ Does the treatment plan include follow-up and monitoring?
- ✓ Would another clinician understand today's visit by reading my note?

Liberty's Lesson #6
Your documentation reflects your clinical judgment.
Early in my career, I realized that good documentation is not about protecting yourself after something goes wrong—it is about clearly communicating your thinking while providing the best possible care.

A thoughtful note tells the patient's story, explains your reasoning, and provides a roadmap for future care. It demonstrates professionalism, supports continuity, and reflects the care you put into every clinical decision.

Write every note with the same care you give every patient.

Clinical Reasoning in Action
"But I Asked About Suicide…"

A new PMHNP evaluates a patient with worsening depression. During the interview, the patient denies suicidal thoughts, reports sleeping poorly, and agrees to begin treatment with an SSRI. The visit goes well, and the patient schedules a follow-up appointment.

Later that day, the clinician reviews the note and realizes it contains only one sentence about safety:
"Patient denies SI/HI."

Although suicide was discussed, the documentation does not include risk factors, protective factors, the patient's future orientation, or the rationale for outpatient management.

The assessment was appropriate. The documentation was incomplete.

Reflection Questions

What additional information would strengthen this documentation?
How would you document the patient's protective factors?
Why is documenting your clinical reasoning as important as documenting the patient's answers?
If another provider saw this patient tomorrow, would they understand why outpatient treatment was appropriate?

How I Would Think Through This Case

Risk assessment is more than documenting whether a patient answered "yes" or "no" to suicidal thoughts.

It includes evaluating the patient's overall level of risk, identifying protective factors, considering relevant clinical history, and explaining why the chosen treatment setting is appropriate.

Good documentation demonstrates that your clinical decisions were thoughtful, individualized, and based on the information available at the time.

Clinical Pearl: Your note should explain not only **what** you decided, but **why** you decided it.

Chapter 7
Avoiding Common Missteps

"Good judgment often develops from experience—but learning from the experience of others is even better."

Every experienced PMHNP can look back and remember decisions they would make differently today. Fortunately, most mistakes in clinical practice are preventable when we slow down, remain curious, and ask for help when needed.

The goal is not to become a perfect clinician.
The goal is to recognize common pitfalls before they become common habits.

Common Misstep #1: Falling in Love with Your First Diagnosis

It is easy to anchor on the first diagnosis that seems to fit.
Resist that temptation.

Keep your differential diagnosis open until you have gathered enough information. Ask yourself, *"What else could explain these symptoms?"*

The best clinicians are willing to change their minds when new information becomes available.

Common Misstep #2: Prescribing Too Quickly

Many new PMHNPs feel pressure to prescribe during every visit.

Remember what we discussed in the previous chapter:
Medication is one treatment option—not the only treatment option.

Sometimes the best clinical decision is to gather more information, obtain collateral history, recommend psychotherapy, or arrange close follow-up before initiating medication.

Never prescribe simply because you feel pressured to "do something."

Common Misstep #3: Treating Symptoms Instead of Understanding the Cause

Insomnia.
Poor concentration.
Anxiety.

These symptoms can occur in dozens of psychiatric and medical conditions.
Treating the symptom without understanding its cause often leads to unnecessary medications and missed diagnoses.

Always ask *why* the symptom is occurring before deciding *how* to treat it.

Common Misstep #4: Forgetting the Medical Differential

Not every psychiatric symptom originates from a psychiatric disorder.

Medical illnesses, neurological conditions, medications, endocrine disorders, sleep disorders, and substance use can all mimic psychiatric disease.

Never stop thinking like an advanced practice clinician.

Common Misstep #5: Overlooking Substance Use

Patients may not volunteer information about alcohol, cannabis, stimulants, opioids, or other substances unless you ask.

Substance use can complicate diagnosis, alter treatment response, and increase safety risks.

Screen routinely and without judgment.

Common Misstep #6: Underestimating the Value of Follow-Up

The initial treatment decision is only the beginning.

Follow-up visits allow you to assess response, monitor adverse effects, refine your diagnosis, and strengthen the therapeutic relationship.

Good outcomes depend on ongoing assessment—not just good initial decisions.

Common Misstep #7: Trying to Know Everything

One of the fastest paths to burnout is believing you must have every answer.
You will not.
Neither do experienced clinicians.

Medicine changes constantly, and psychiatry continues to evolve.

The strongest clinicians remain lifelong students.

Looking Ahead

Avoiding pitfalls is part of becoming a safe clinician.
Equally important is learning how to communicate effectively—not only with patients, but also with families, colleagues, therapists, pharmacists, and primary care providers.

Communication is one of your most powerful clinical tools, and that is where we will turn next.

Mentor's Corner

When you are uncertain, slow down.
Review the chart.
Revisit your differential diagnosis.
Consult a colleague.
Thoughtful clinicians are remembered for their judgment—not their speed.

Quick Checklist

- ✓ *Before finalizing a diagnosis or treatment plan, ask yourself:*
- ✓ *Have I considered reasonable alternative diagnoses?*
- ✓ *Have I ruled out medical, neurological, or substance-related causes?*
- ✓ *Am I prescribing because it's clinically appropriate—or because I feel pressured?*
- ✓ *Do I have enough information to make today's decision safely?*
- ✓ *Is my follow-up plan appropriate for this patient's level of risk?*

Liberty's Lesson #7
Your greatest clinical asset is not intelligence—it is humility.

Some of the best lessons I. learned came from asking questions, seeking consultation, and occasionally realizing that my first impression was not my best one.

Psychiatry teaches us to remain curious.

Patients do not benefit from clinicians who always appear certain.
They benefit from clinicians who think carefully, listen deeply, and are willing to reconsider when new information emerges.
Humility is not a limitation.
It is one of the hallmarks of clinical excellence.

Clinical Reasoning in Action
"It's Just Anxiety…"

A 29-year-old woman presents with worsening anxiety, restlessness, poor concentration, and insomnia. She reports feeling "on edge" for several months and asks whether she should start medication for anxiety.

At first glance, Generalized Anxiety Disorder seems like a reasonable diagnosis.

As you continue the interview, she mentions an unintentional 15-pound weight loss despite an increased appetite, frequent palpitations, heat intolerance, and a fine tremor that she assumed was caused by stress.

Instead of immediately prescribing an anxiolytic, you recommend a medical evaluation, including thyroid function testing, while continuing your psychiatric assessment.

A week later, her laboratory results reveal significant hyperthyroidism.

Reflection Questions

What additional medical conditions can mimic anxiety?
What history or physical findings prompted further evaluation?
Would prescribing medication immediately have addressed the underlying problem?
How can collaboration with primary care improve patient outcomes?

How I Would Think Through This Case

Psychiatric symptoms do not always originate from psychiatric illness.

Before assigning a psychiatric diagnosis, I ask myself whether a medical condition, medication, substance, or neurological disorder could better explain the presentation.

In this case, the patient's physical symptoms broadened the differential diagnosis and prompted appropriate medical evaluation before initiating psychiatric treatment.

Treating presumed anxiety alone might have delayed the diagnosis of an important endocrine disorder.

Clinical Pearl: One of the safest habits you can develop is asking, *"Could this be medical before I conclude it is psychiatric?"*

Chapter 8
Protecting Your License—and Yourself

"Your license is one of the most valuable things you will ever earn. Protect it with the same care you give your patients."

Becoming a PMHNP is a tremendous accomplishment. Protecting your license is a lifelong responsibility.

Most disciplinary actions do not occur because clinicians intentionally harm patients. They often result from poor documentation, inadequate follow-up, boundary issues, prescribing without appropriate assessment, or failing to recognize when additional help is needed.

Fortunately, many of these situations are preventable.

Practice Within Your Competence

One of the most important professional responsibilities is recognizing the limits of your knowledge and experience.

You do not have to know everything.

If a patient presents with a condition outside your comfort level, seek consultation, review current evidence, or refer when appropriate.

Patients are safest when clinicians recognize both their strengths and their limitations.

Clinical Pearl

Knowing when to ask for help is a sign of clinical maturity—not weakness.

Maintain Professional Boundaries

Psychiatry often involves caring for patients during some of the most vulnerable moments of their lives. Strong therapeutic relationships are essential, but professional boundaries must always remain clear.

Avoid situations that could compromise objectivity or create conflicts of interest.

Think carefully before accepting gifts, communicating through personal social media accounts, or sharing unnecessary personal information.
Healthy boundaries protect both you and your patients.

Prescribe Thoughtfully

Controlled substances deserve special attention.

Before prescribing, ask yourself:
Is there a clear clinical indication?
Have I reviewed the patient's history and current medications?
Have I assessed for substance use or misuse?
Have I reviewed the Prescription Drug Monitoring Program (PDMP), when applicable?
Have I documented my clinical reasoning?

Never allow time pressure or patient expectations to replace sound clinical judgment.

Communication Prevents Problems
Many misunderstandings can be prevented through clear communication.

Explain your diagnosis.
Discuss the expected benefits and risks of treatment.
Review follow-up plans.
Encourage questions.

Patients are more likely to trust your decisions when they understand the reasoning behind them—even when the answer is "not today."

Never Stop Learning
Psychiatry continues to evolve.

New medications become available.
Practice guidelines change.
Research expands our understanding of mental illness.

Protecting your license means protecting your knowledge. Make continuing education, consultation, and self-reflection part of your professional routine.

Your patients deserve a clinician who continues to grow.

Looking Ahead
A successful career is measured by more than clinical knowledge.

It is also measured by professional fulfillment, resilience, and maintaining your passion for caring for others.

In our final chapter, we will discuss how to build a meaningful, sustainable career as a PMHNP.

Mentor's Corner
Protecting your license is not about practicing defensively.
It is about practicing thoughtfully.

When you consistently place patient safety, ethical decision-making, and sound clinical judgment at the center of your practice, you are also protecting yourself.

Quick Checklist
Before making an important clinical decision, ask yourself:

- ✓ *Am I practicing within my current level of competence?*
- ✓ *Have I documented my clinical reasoning?*
- ✓ *Have I communicated the risks, benefits, and follow-up plan clearly?*
- ✓ *Have I considered consultation or referral if needed?*
- ✓ *Would I be comfortable explaining this decision to a colleague—or to a licensing board if necessary?*

Liberty's Lesson #8
Your reputation is built one patient at a time.

Patients may forget the exact medication you prescribed or the wording of your treatment plan, but they will remember how you treated them.

Be respectful.
Be honest.
Be prepared.
Be willing to admit when you do not know something and take the time to find the answer.

Professional integrity is not demonstrated during your best days. It is demonstrated during your most difficult ones—when you are tired, behind schedule, or faced with a challenging decision.

Your license allows you to practice.
Your integrity earns the trust that makes your practice meaningful.

Clinical Reasoning in Action
"Can You Make an Exception?"

A 38-year-old established patient calls the office late on a Friday afternoon requesting an early refill of a controlled medication. He explains that he is leaving town for the weekend and forgot to request the refill sooner. He becomes increasingly frustrated when told that an early refill may not be appropriate.

The schedule is full, staff members are waiting to leave, and you feel pressure to resolve the situation quickly.

Granting the refill would be easy.
Taking a few extra minutes to review the chart, check the PDMP, review previous refill dates, and document your decision would take more time—but it would also support safe prescribing.

Reflection Questions
What additional information would you obtain before making a decision?
How would you respond if the patient became upset?
How can you balance empathy with appropriate prescribing practices?
What documentation would support your decision, regardless of the outcome?

How I Would Think Through This Case
Requests made under pressure deserve thoughtful evaluation—not automatic approval or automatic denial.

I would review the patient's treatment history, medication agreement (if applicable), PDMP data, refill history, and any documented concerns regarding misuse or diversion. I would then communicate my decision respectfully, explain the rationale, and document both the clinical reasoning and the discussion.

Maintaining professional boundaries sometimes means saying "no" when it is clinically appropriate.

Patients may not always agree with your decision, but they should always understand that it was made with fairness, consistency, and their safety in mind.

Clinical Pearl: The easiest decision is not always the safest one. When you feel pressured to act quickly, that is often the moment to slow down and think.

Chapter 9
Your Career Is a Marathon, Not a Sprint

"A successful career is not measured by how much you accomplish in your first year—it is measured by how much you continue to grow throughout your lifetime."

Congratulations.
If you have read this far, you have taken an important step toward becoming not just a competent PMHNP, but a thoughtful one.

Your first job will teach you many things. Some days you will leave the office feeling confident. Other days you will replay conversations in your mind, wondering whether you could have asked one more question or chosen a different treatment plan.

That is part of becoming a clinician.
Growth does not happen because you never make mistakes. Growth happens because you are willing to reflect, learn, and continue moving forward.

Never Stop Learning

One of the greatest privileges of psychiatry is that there is always something new to learn.

New research.
New medications.
New approaches to psychotherapy.
New technologies.

Every patient you meet will teach you something that no textbook ever could.
Protect your curiosity. It will become one of your greatest professional strengths.

Clinical Pearl
The day you believe you have learned everything is the day you stop growing as a clinician.

Find Your Professional Community

Medicine is a team sport.

Stay connected with classmates, mentors, former preceptors, psychiatrists, psychologists, therapists, pharmacists, nurses, and primary care colleagues.
Attend conferences.
Join professional organizations.
Participate in case discussions.

Teach when you have something to share.
Learn when someone has something to teach you.

Your professional community will challenge you, encourage you, and remind you that you are never alone in this journey.

Discover Your Passion
Psychiatry offers countless opportunities.

You may discover a passion for:

- Child and adolescent psychiatry
- Geriatric psychiatry
- Addiction medicine
- Forensic psychiatry
- Women's mental health
- Sleep medicine
- Neuromodulation
- Research
- Teaching
- Leadership
- Advocacy
- Entrepreneurship

Your career does not have to look like anyone else's.
Allow it to evolve as your interests and experiences grow.

Take Care of Yourself
You cannot pour from an empty cup.

Psychiatric practice is deeply rewarding, but it can also be emotionally demanding.

Protect your own well-being.
Maintain relationships outside of work.
Take vacations.
Celebrate your successes.

Learn from difficult days without carrying them home.
Seeking support for yourself is not a sign of weakness. It is part of being a healthy healthcare professional.

Remember Why You Started
There will be busy clinic days.
Prior authorizations.
Documentation.
Insurance requirements.
Administrative responsibilities.

Do not let those challenges cause you to forget why you chose psychiatry.

Every day, you have the opportunity to reduce suffering, restore hope, and change the trajectory of someone's life.

Never underestimate the difference your presence can make.

A Final Thought

One day, you will mentor a student.
You will answer questions from a new graduate.
You will reassure someone who wonders if they are ready.
And you will smile because you will remember asking those same questions yourself.

When that day comes, I hope you will share not only your knowledge but also your kindness, humility, and encouragement.

Our profession grows stronger when we invest in one another.

Thank you for allowing me to be part of your journey.

I have every confidence that you will make a meaningful difference in the lives of your patients and in the future of our profession.

Welcome to the remarkable community of Psychiatric Mental Health Nurse Practitioners.

Your journey is just beginning.

Mentor's Corner

Never compare the beginning of your career to someone else's twenty years of experience.

Every expert was once a beginner.
Keep learning.
Keep growing.
Keep showing up.

Quick Checklist

As you move forward in your career, ask yourself regularly:

- ✓ *Am I continuing to learn?*
- ✓ *Am I seeking mentorship and offering it to others?*
- ✓ *Am I caring for my own well-being?*
- ✓ *Am I practicing with integrity and compassion?*
- ✓ *Am I becoming the clinician I hoped to be?*

Liberty's Lesson #9
Success is not defined by titles, awards, or the number of patients you see.

It is reflected in the lives you touch, the trust you earn, and the legacy you leave behind.

Throughout my career, I have learned that the most fulfilling opportunities often began with simply saying "yes" to learning something new. Those experiences led me to become a clinician, educator, researcher, speaker, entrepreneur, and mentor. None of those roles were part of a master plan—they grew naturally from a willingness to remain curious and embrace new challenges. I attend conferences regularly. I present posters in conventions. I do podium presentations. I continue to read psychiatry and NP journals. I am active in my NP associations.

As your career unfolds, do not be afraid to explore new paths. Your professional journey may take you places you never imagined.

Most importantly, remember that behind every diagnosis is a person who has trusted you with their story.
Honor that trust every single day.

Reflection Questions
Have you ever compared yourself to a more experienced clinician?
What does lifelong learning look like in your career?
Who will you turn to when you need guidance?
How will you mentor someone else in the future?

Epilogue
Now Go Take Care of Someone

When you first opened this book, you were probably looking for answers.
How do I know if I'm ready?
What if I make a mistake?
How do experienced PMHNPs think?

I hope you have found some of those answers in these pages.
But I also hope you have discovered something even more important.

No book can teach you everything.
No mentor can prepare you for every patient.
No degree marks the end of learning.

Your education did not end when you graduated. It did not end when you passed your board certification. And it will not end after your first year in practice.

Each patient you meet will become one of your teachers.
Some will teach you about resilience.
Others will teach you about heartbreak.
Some will remind you that healing takes time.
Others will remind you that hope can return even when it seems impossible.

If you remain curious, humble, and compassionate, your patients will continue to shape you into the clinician you are meant to become.

There will be days when you leave the office feeling proud of the difference you made.

There will also be days when you will wonder if you could have done more.
Those moments are part of every meaningful career.

Learn from them, but do not let them define you.
Celebrate your successes.
Reflect on your challenges.
Forgive yourself when you are imperfect.
Then return the next day ready to care for another person.

Never forget that behind every diagnosis is a human being with fears, dreams, relationships, disappointments, and hopes. Long after patients forget the names of their medications or the details of a treatment plan, many will remember how you made them feel.

Be the clinician who listens before speaking.
Be the clinician who treats every patient with dignity and respect.
Be the clinician who is not afraid to say, "I don't know, but I'll find out."
Be the clinician who continues learning long after the diploma is framed on the wall.

One day, you will look back and realize that the new graduate who once questioned every decision has become the colleague others seek for guidance.
When that day comes, I hope you will remember your own beginning.

Answer the phone when a new graduate calls with a question.
Encourage the student who feels overwhelmed.
Share your knowledge generously.
Our profession grows stronger every time we lift someone else.

Thank you for allowing me to be part of your journey.

With gratitude,

Liberty Olive RB Macias, DNP, APRN, PMHNP-BC

Before you close this book, I would like to leave you with one final piece of advice.

Protect your professional relationships.

Psychiatry is a remarkably small community. Throughout your career, you will cross paths with former classmates, preceptors, collaborating physicians, nurses, therapists, psychologists, pharmacists, social workers, administrators, and students more often than you can imagine. Today's classmate may become tomorrow's colleague. Today's preceptor may write a recommendation for a future opportunity. Today's student may one day become your coworker.

Treat everyone with professionalism, respect, and kindness.

Do not burn bridges.

Disagreements will happen. Jobs will change. People will move on to different organizations and different roles. Leave every position with integrity, gratitude, and professionalism. Your reputation will often arrive before you do.

Seek mentors throughout your career, but also strive to become the kind of colleague others trust and enjoy working with. Celebrate the success of others.

Share what you have learned. Ask questions without embarrassment, and offer guidance <u>without</u> arrogance.

No one builds a meaningful career alone.

The relationships you cultivate throughout your professional journey will become one of your greatest sources of wisdom, encouragement, opportunity, and lifelong friendship.

Never underestimate the power of being known—not only as an excellent clinician, but also as an excellent colleague.

www.ingramcontent.com/pod-product-compliance
Lightning Source LLC
LaVergne TN
LVHW100201061126
851857LV00010B/355
* 9 7 9 8 9 9 7 3 2 1 5 1 2 *